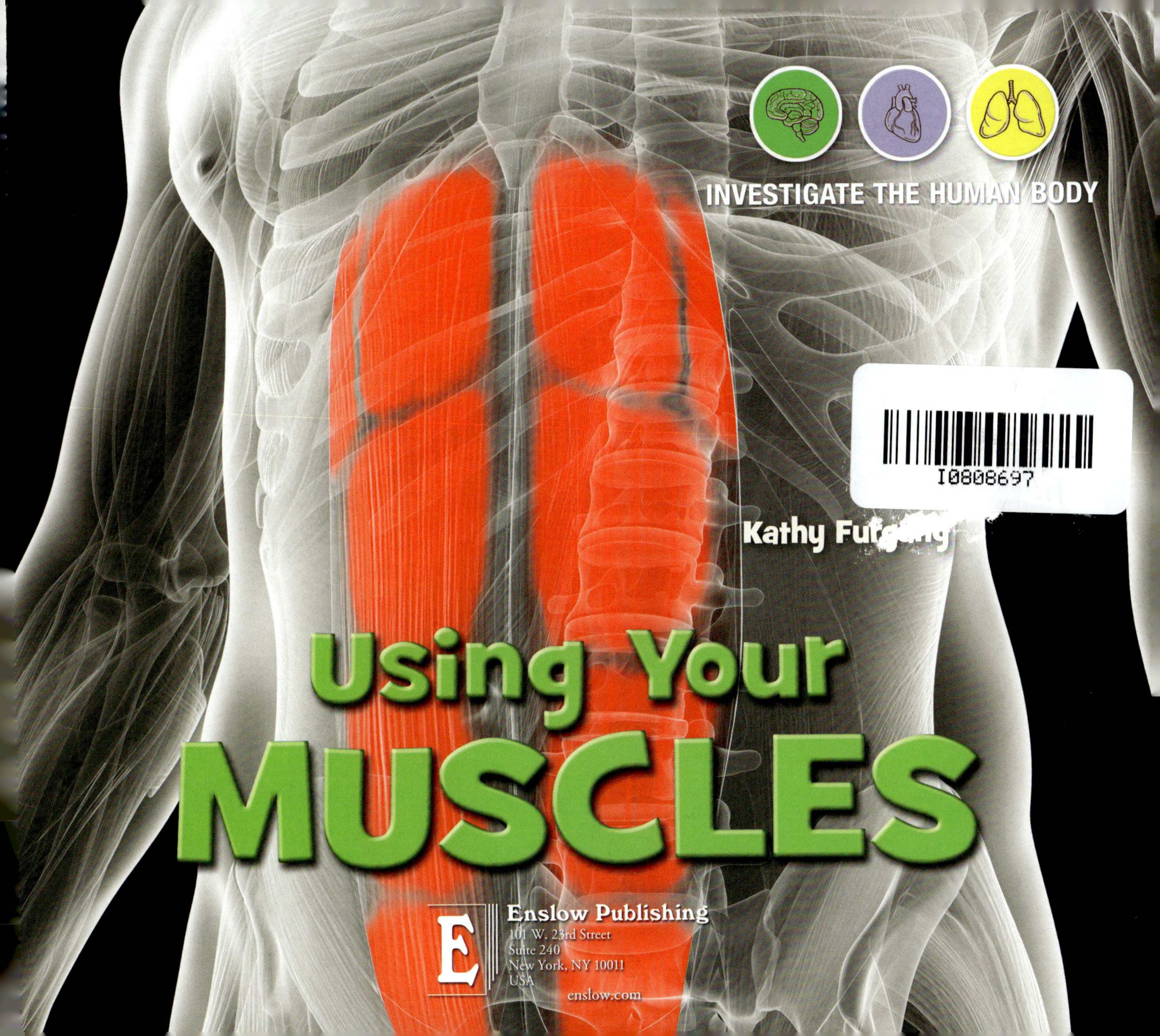

INVESTIGATE THE HUMAN BODY

Kathy Fu[illegible]

Using Your MUSCLES

Enslow Publishing
101 W. 23rd Street
Suite 240
New York, NY 10011
USA
enslow.com

Words to Know

contract To become shorter and tighter.

fiber A thin structure shaped like a thread.

inherited Passed on at birth.

involuntary Without being controlled or thought about.

nerve A bundle of fibers that carries messages to and from the brain.

nutrient Something that animals and plants take in to live and grow.

oxygen A gas in the air and body that is needed for living and breathing.

tendon Flexible fiber that connects muscles to bone.

voluntary Able to be controlled.

Contents

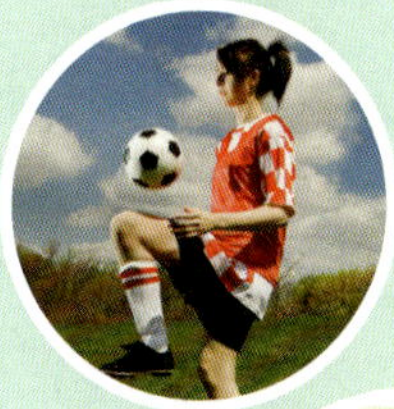

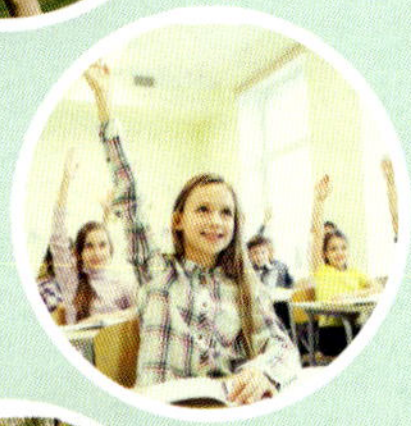

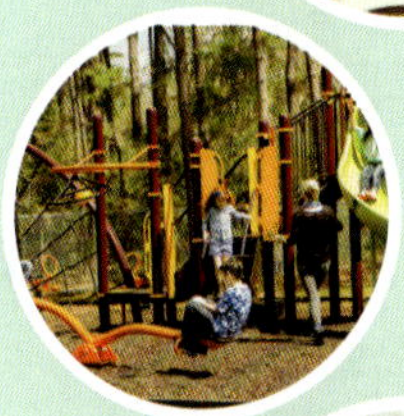

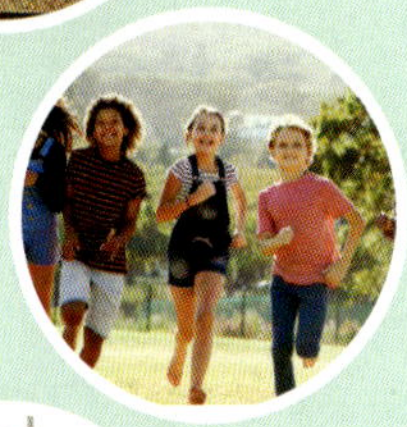

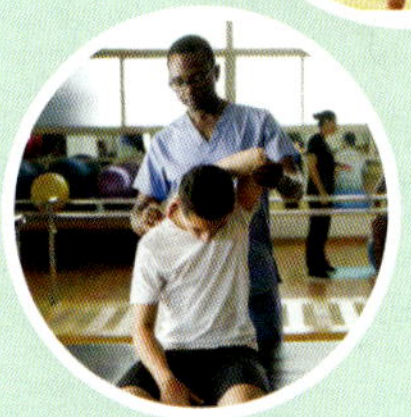

How We Use Our Muscles

When someone says "**make a muscle,**" what do you do? You hold up your arm and flex it until it bulges as much as possible. But did you know you are "making muscles" with every move you make? Your muscles help you to do just about anything!

Think about a few of the things you do in a day. You stand. You walk. You wave. You digest food. All of these actions depend on muscles. You raise your hand to answer your teacher's question. This simple act requires many messages back and forth from your brain to your muscles. Just imagine the number of messages needed for you to write your name or use a video game controller!

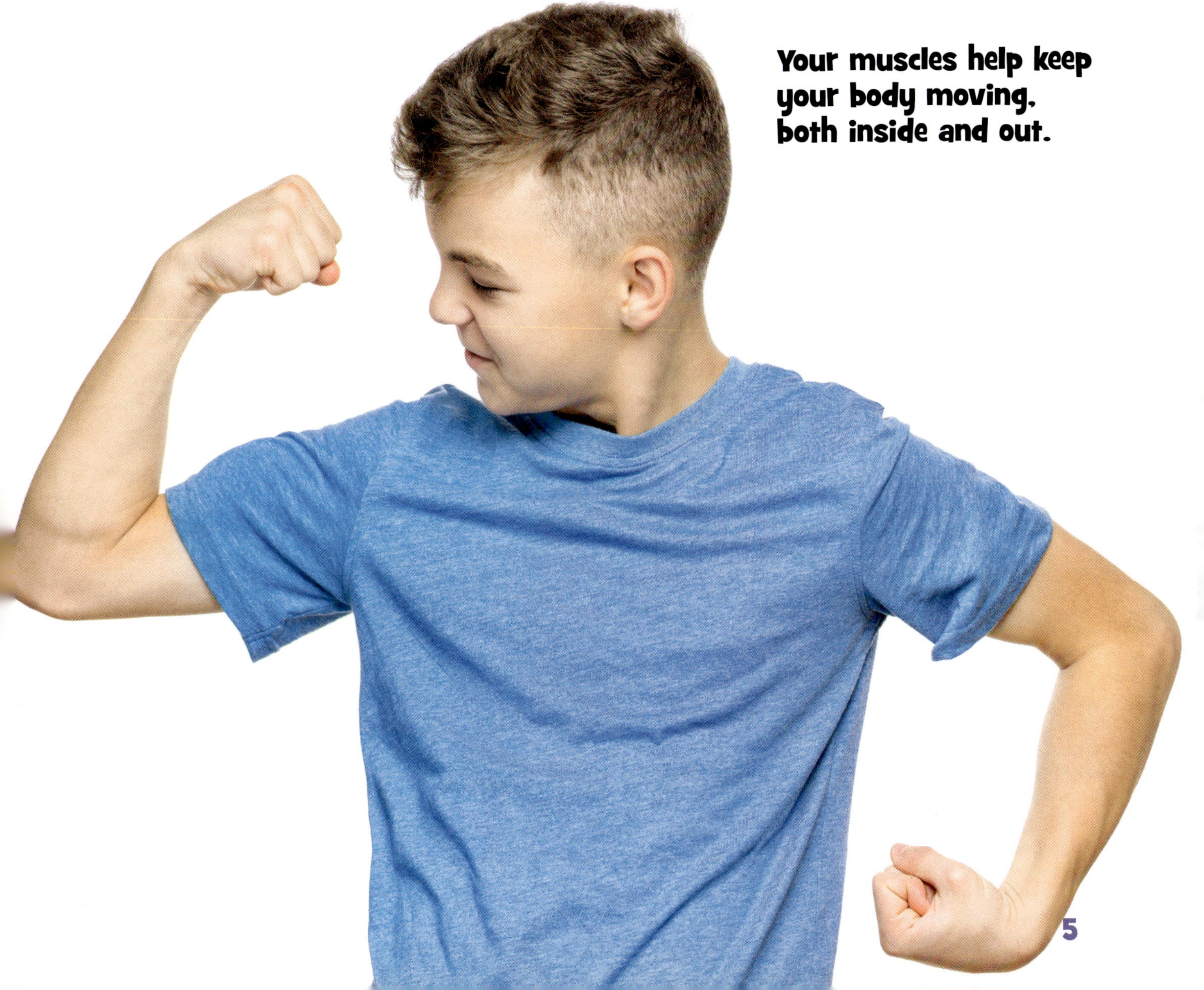

Your muscles help keep your body moving, both inside and out.

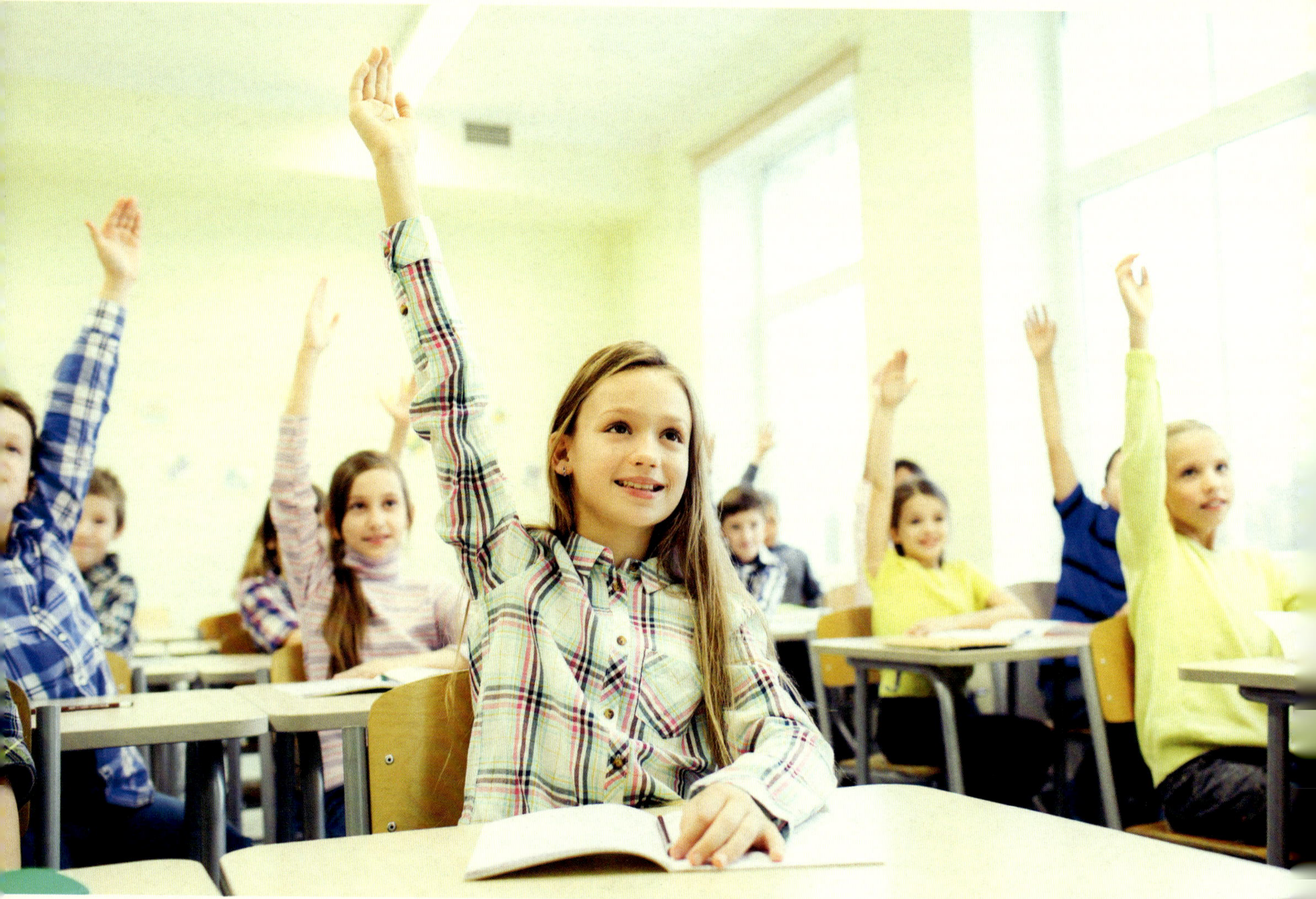

Simply lifting your hand in the air involves many muscle movements.

Bending your knee requires muscles in your thigh and lower leg.

Working in Pairs

Muscles are long, thin bundles of **fiber**. Inside these fibers are **nerves** that communicate with the rest of your body. Nerves let you know when you are in pain. They can also let you know when you have moved or lifted as much as you possibly can.

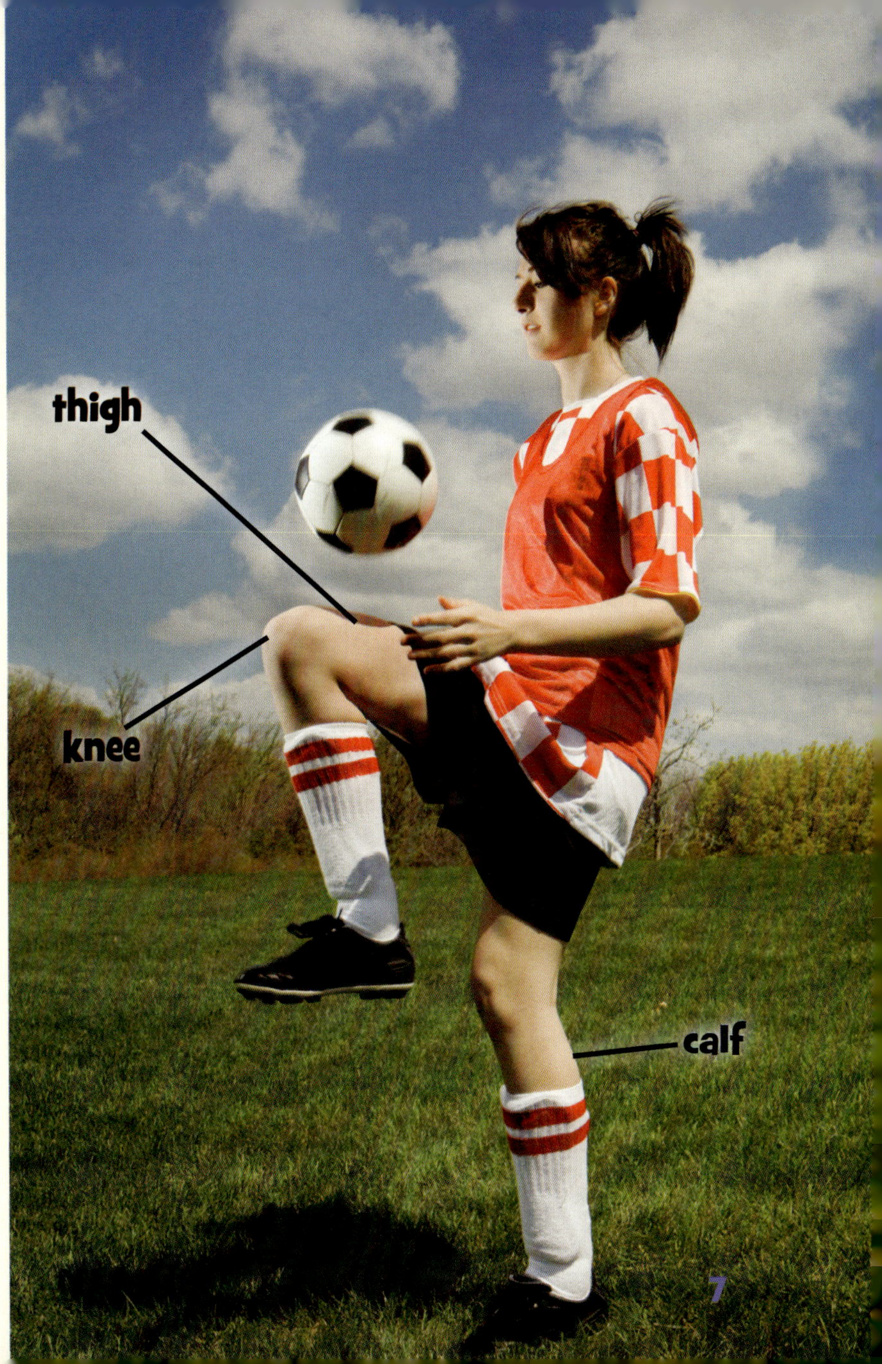

Many Muscles

Your body has more than 650 muscles that connect to your skeleton.

Muscles work together in pairs to allow your body to move. When one muscle **contracts**, or tightens, another one relaxes to allow space for the movement. Think about bending your knee, for example. Muscles behind your leg contract while the ones in front of it relax.

Types of Muscles

There are three different types of muscles in your body. The ones that help you move are called skeletal muscles. These muscles do exactly what you might think. They connect to the bones of your skeleton! Skeletal muscles allow all of your different body parts to move. This kind of muscle movement is **voluntary**.

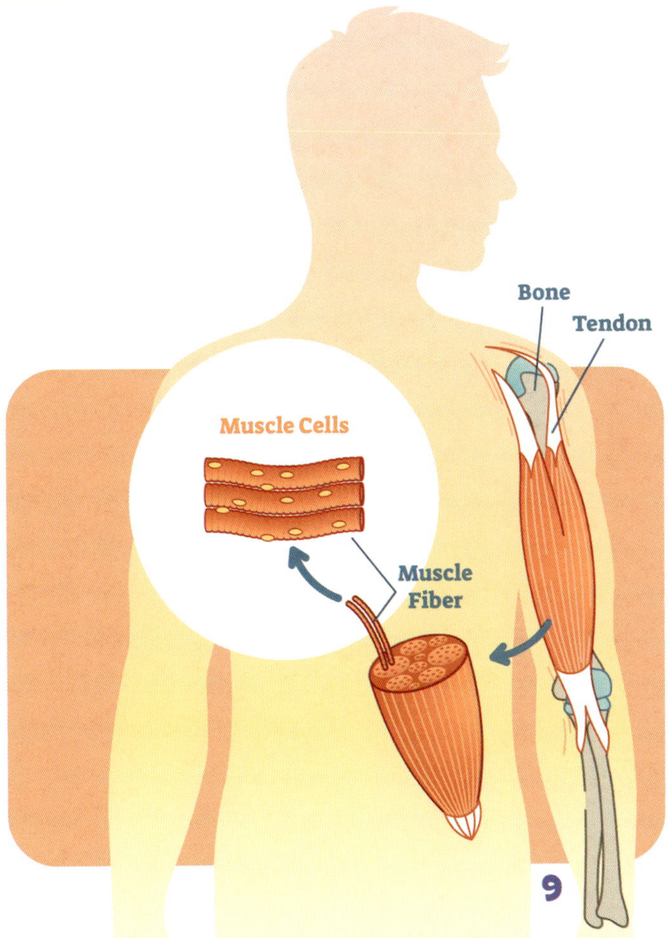

Muscle fibers inside muscles connect to tendons. The tendons connect to bone.

That means that you can control and think about the muscles when you move them. Flexible fibers called tendons connect the muscles to bones.

Wrapped inside muscles are long muscle fibers. They wrap together in tight bundles that control your movement. Inside the muscles are also tiny tubes called blood vessels. Their job is to move blood around your body. The muscles in your body make up about 40 percent of the weight of your entire body.

Shake Like a Leaf

Shivering is a kind of involuntary muscle movement. Your body shivers to try to control reactions to cold, fear, or excitement.

Muscles control the actions of your heart, stomach, and intestines.

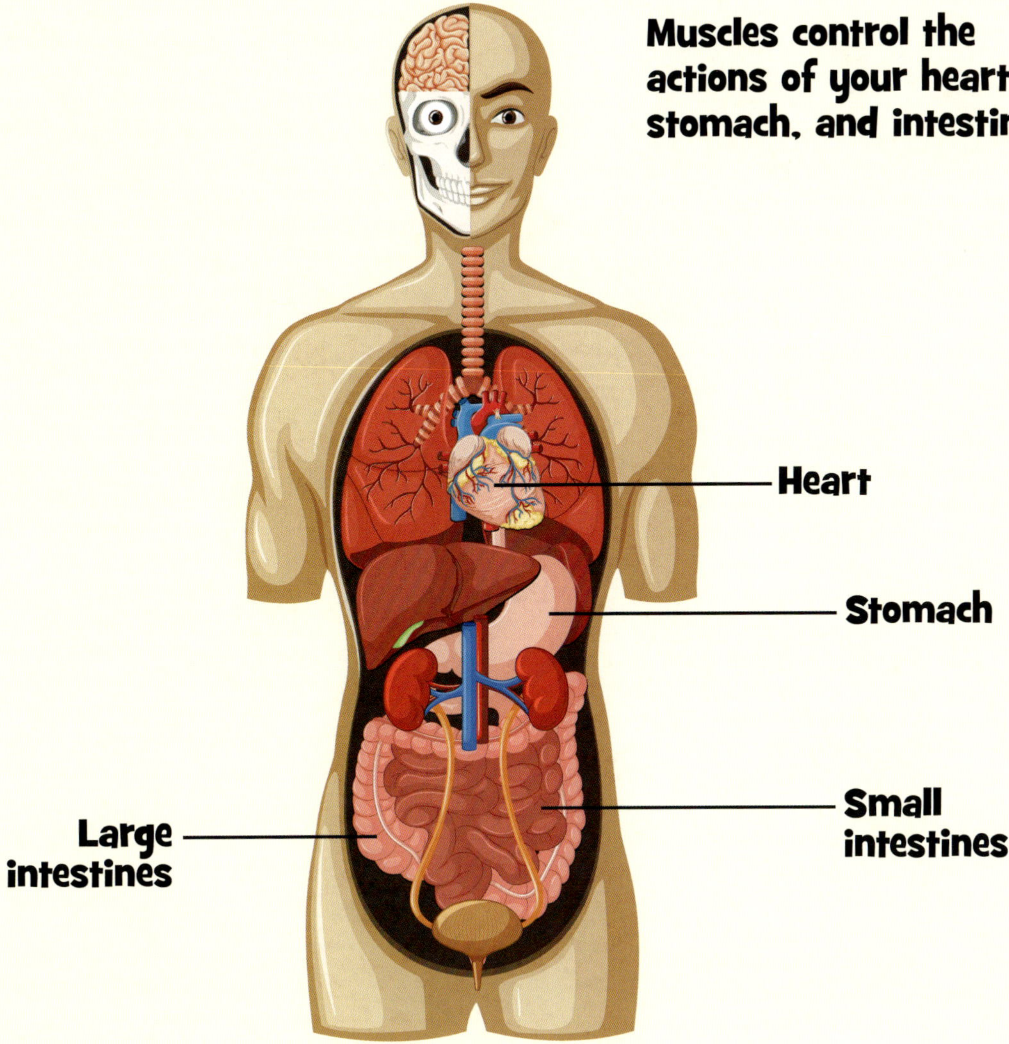

More Muscle Types

Besides skeletal muscle, your body has two other types of muscle. One type is called smooth muscle. It is also called involuntary muscle. These muscles cause movements that you cannot control, like the actions of your body's organs. Movements in your gut, stomach, and throat are controlled by smooth muscles. The muscles expand and contract on their own to allow movement. They are not attached to bone.

The third type of muscle is cardiac muscle. Cardiac muscle's only job is to control the beating of your heart. This repeating action pumps blood through your entire body.

The Muscular System

All of the muscles in your body make up the muscular system. Your muscular system works along with your skeletal system. You could not move without both systems working together. For every movement of the skeleton, muscles move with it.

Long bones such as the legs and arms are

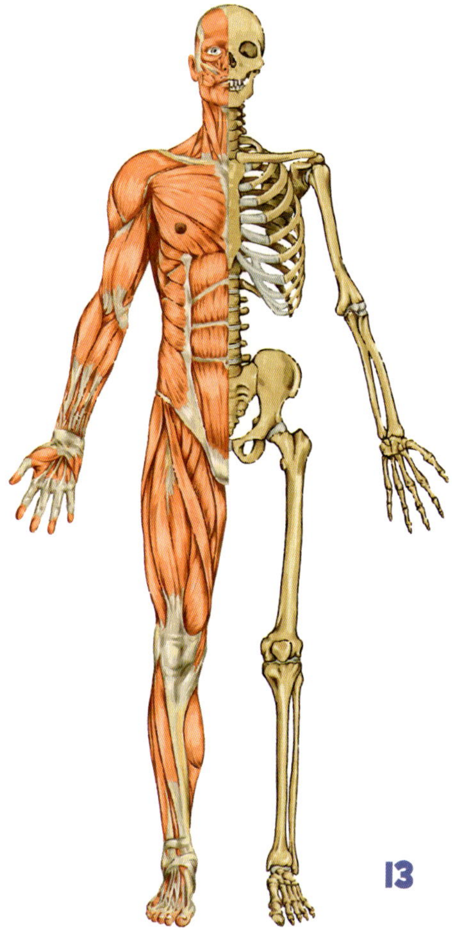

Muscles cover every bone in your body, including your ribs and back.

covered with the longest muscle fibers. They must be strong enough to lift and stretch. On the other hand, bones in your fingers and toes are covered with shorter, thinner muscles. The movement of your muscles helps send blood and **nutrients** around your body. These make you healthy and strong.

A Smooth Operation

Your muscular system is not just important for moving. The bundles of nerve fibers keep your body systems working right. The connections between your heart muscles and blood vessels bring **oxygen** and nutrients through your entire body. The body needs oxygen for energy and growth.

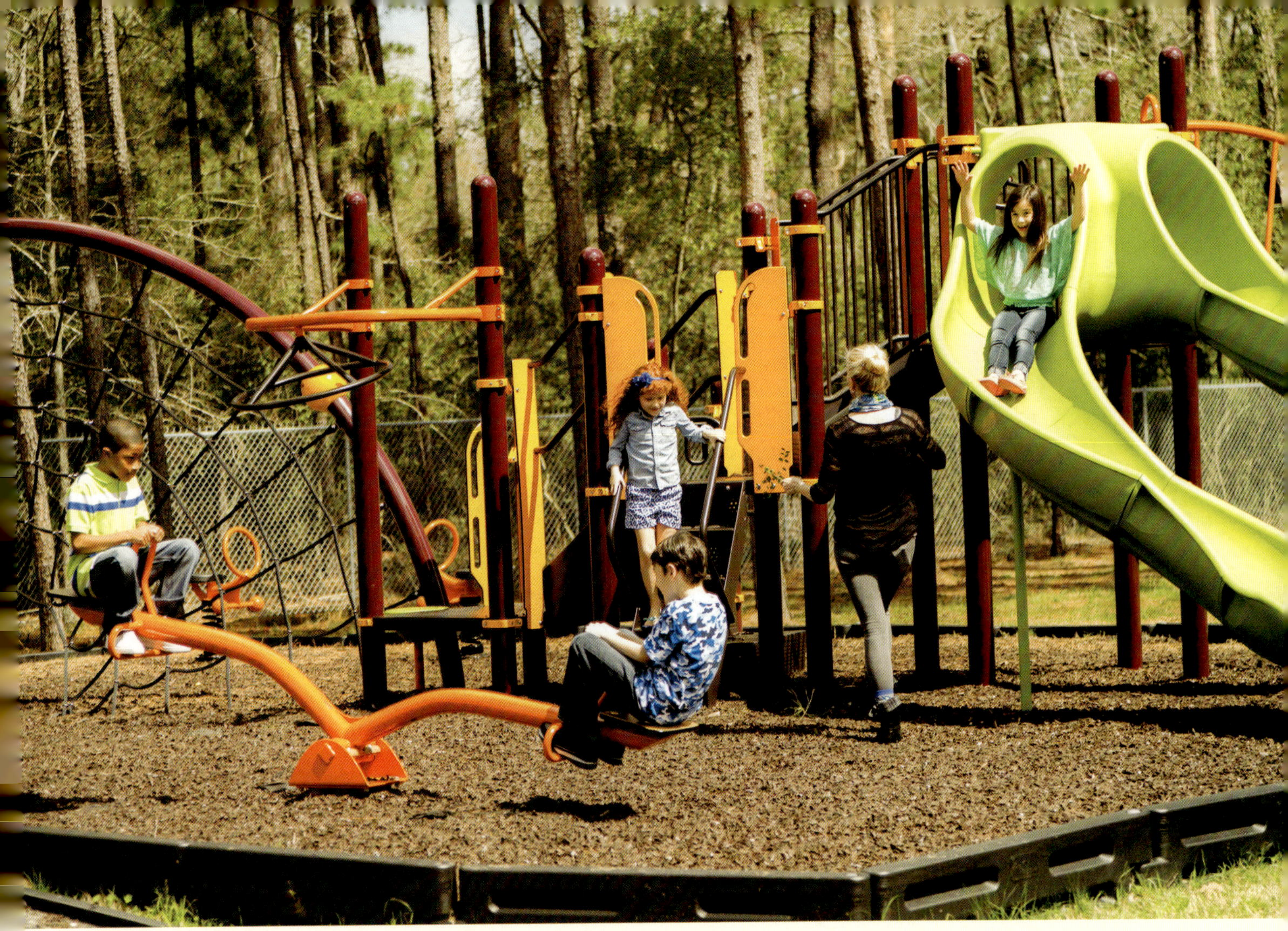

Even just a little movement is enough to pump blood to your muscles.

Say Cheese!

You use muscles in your face to both smile and frown.

So, the more you move around, the more chance your body has to pump fresh blood and oxygen to your body parts. This make you feel strong and alert. If you stayed in one position all day your body would begin to feel uncomfortable and weak. Muscle movements and blood flow help keep your body in shape.

Treat Your Muscles Right

A healthy body starts with healthy connections between the brain and body. Certain diseases weaken muscles or keep them from acting like they should. Some diseases affect the way skeletal muscles work. Polio is a muscular disease caused by a virus. Other muscular diseases are **inherited**. That means they are passed on at birth.

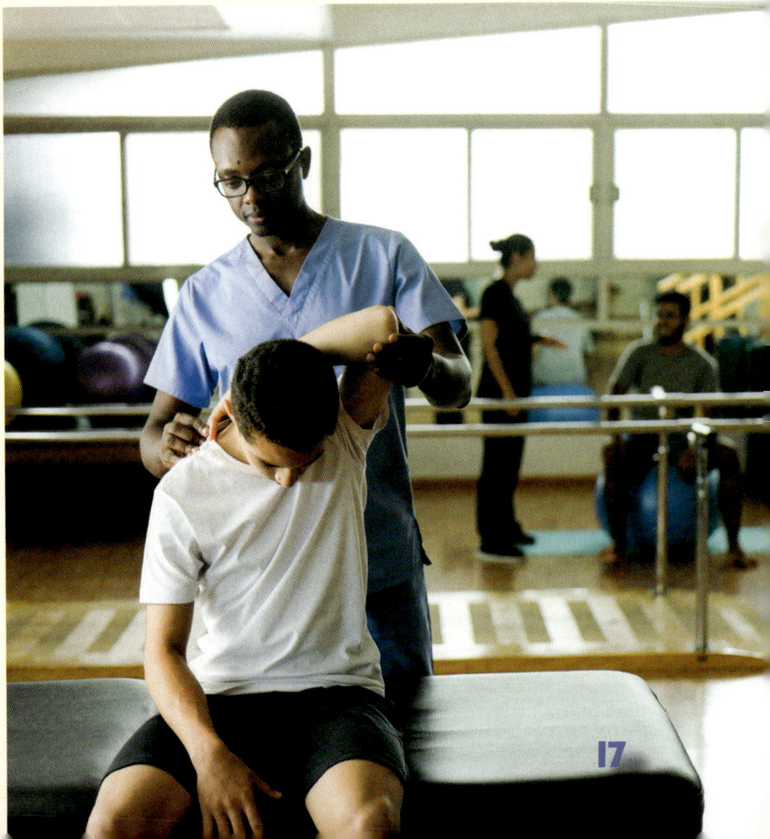

Physical therapists work with patients who have injuries or diseases of the muscles.

Some illnesses keep a person from using muscles correctly. There are ways to treat these illnesses. Medicine or therapy can help control the disease. Scientists study diseases to learn more about how the muscular and skeletal systems work together.

Eat Right for Muscle Health

How can you keep your muscles strong and healthy? It is important to have a good diet. The foods you eat affect all parts of your body. Foods that are high in protein help build muscles and keep them working properly. Eggs, lean meats, beans, and nuts are good sources of proteins.

Carbohydrates are also good for restoring and repairing muscles that are tired or damaged. Potatoes, rice, and many vegetables have carbohydrates. Some fats even help keep muscles strong and healthy.

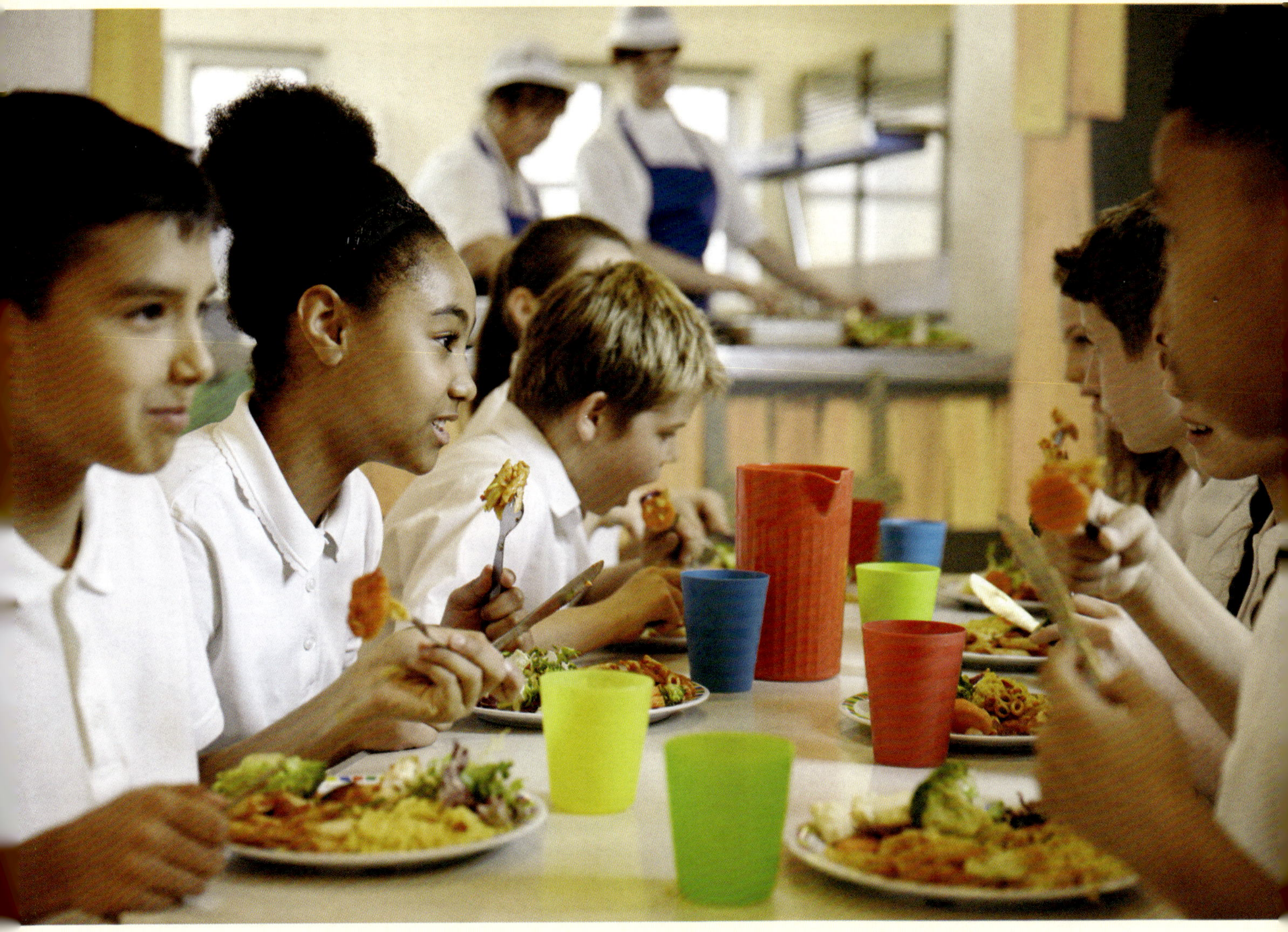

A mix of proteins, carbohydrates, and fats can build strong muscles.

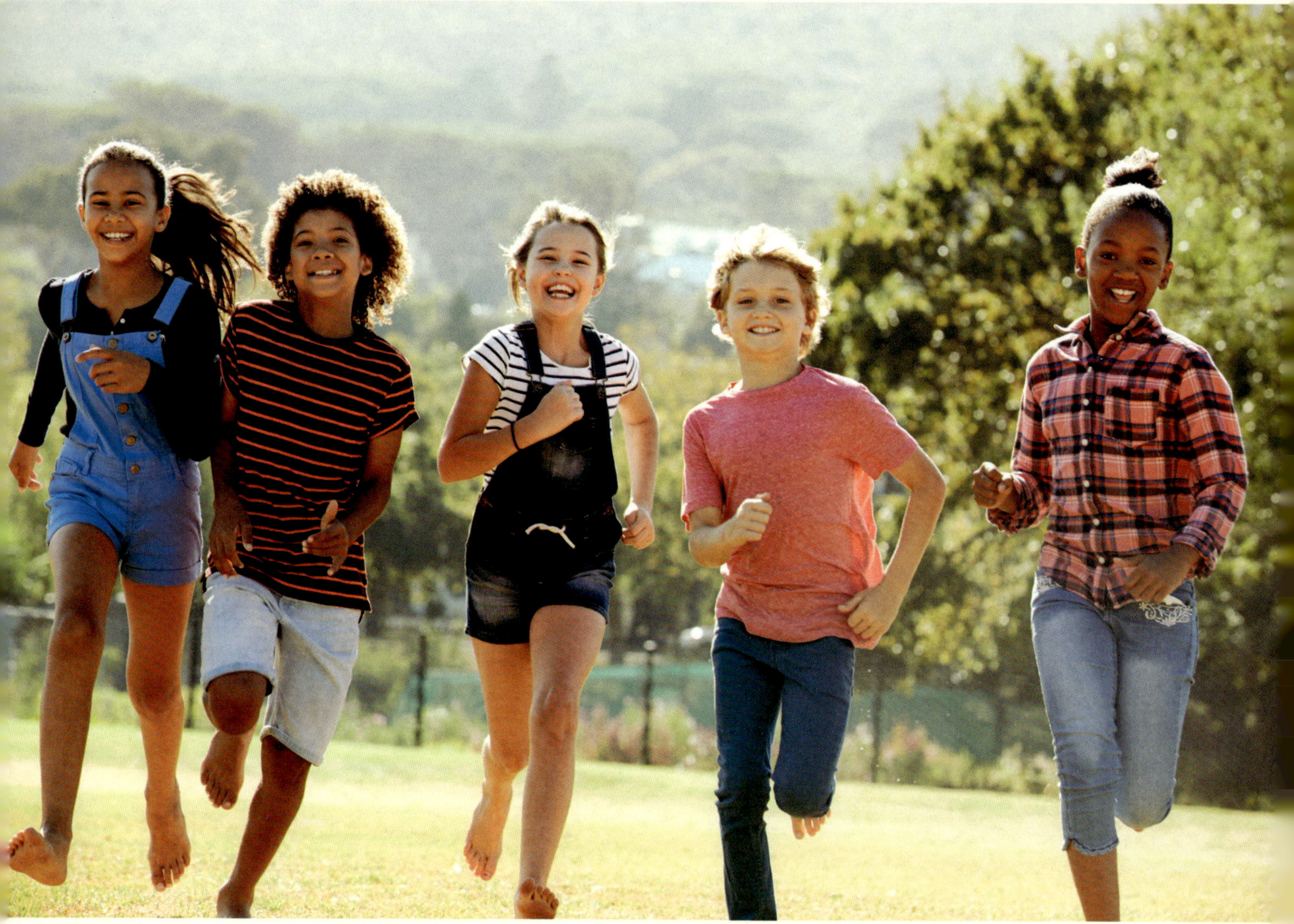

Exercising brings more oxygen to your muscles.

Get Moving

Taking just one step forward uses about 200 muscles in your body.

Use It or Lose It

One of the best things to do for muscle health is exercise. You may have heard the phrase "use it or lose it." This is very true when it comes to exercise and muscles. People who do not exercise can lose most of their body's muscle strength by the time they are 65 years old.

Exercise helps more than just your muscles. It also helps your brain. Exercise makes the brain think more clearly. It also releases chemicals in the brain that make you feel happy. With all these benefits, there is no reason not to exercise your muscles to keep them strong and healthy.

Activity: Simon Says "Flex It!"

Work in a group. Assign one person to play the part of "Simon" in a game of Simon Says.

1. Have Simon name different muscles and ask the group to flex them. For example, "Simon Says flex your foot." "Simon says flex your arm."
2. The rest of the group flexes the muscle that Simon points out.
3. Players are "out" by flexing muscles when Simon does not first say "Simon says…"
4. When Simon has named five muscles in a row, players attempt to remember and call back all of the muscles that were used during the game.

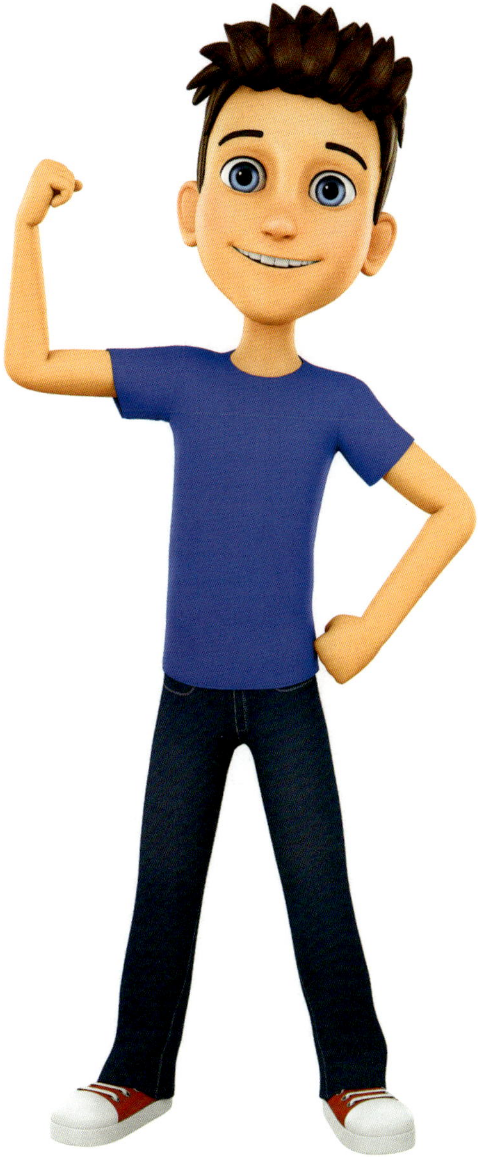

Learn More

Books

Baby Professor. *Human Body Book: Introduction to the Muscular System*. Newark, DE: Speedy Publishing, 2016.

Farndon, John. *Stickmen's Guide to Your Mighty Muscles and Bones*. Minneapolis, MN: Hungry Tomato, 2017.

Heavenrich, Sue. *How Muscles Work*. Vero Beach, FL: Rourke, 2018.

Websites

BAM! Body and Mind

www.cdc.gov/bam/index.html

This website includes information, games, and quizzes about kids' exercise, safety, nutrition, and more.

DK Find Out!

www.dkfindout.com/uk/human-body/

Visit an interactive website all about the human body.

Index

Published in 2020 by Enslow Publishing, LLC
101 W. 23rd Street, Suite 240, New York, NY 10011

Copyright © 2020 by Enslow Publishing, LLC.
All rights reserved.

No part of this book may be reproduced by any means without the written permission of the publisher.

Library of Congress Cataloging-in-Publication Data
Names: Furgang, Kathy, author.
Title: Using your muscles / Kathy Furgang.
Description: New York : Enslow Publishing, 2020. | Series: Investigate the human body | Audience: Grade K-4. | Includes bibliographical references and index.
Identifiers: LCCN 2019015459| ISBN 9781978513037 (library bound) | ISBN 9781978513013 (paperback) | ISBN 9781978513020 (6 pack)
Subjects: LCSH: Muscles--Juvenile literature.
Classification: LCC QP321 .F87 2020 | DDC 612.7/4--dc23
LC record available at https://lccn.loc.gov/2019015459

Printed in the United States of America

To Our Readers: We have done our best to make sure all website addresses in this book were active and appropriate when we went to press. However, the author and the publisher have no control over and assume no liability for the material available on those websites or on any websites they may link to. Any comments or suggestions can be sent by email to customerservice@enslow.com.

Photos Credits: Using Your Muscles – Research by Bruce Donnola
Cover, p. 1 Sebastian Kaulitzki/Shutterstock.com; pp. 3, 7 © iStockphoto.com/YinYang; pp. 3, 6 Syda Productions/Shutterstock.com; pp. 3, 15 © iStockphoto.com/fstop123; pp. 3, 20 © iStockphoto.com/monkeybusinessimages; pp. 3, 17 © iStockphoto.com/aldomurillo; p. 5 VaLiza/Shutterstock.com; p. 9 VectorMine/Shutterstock.com; p. 11 GraphicsRF/Shutterstock.com; p. 13 stihii/Shutterstock.com; p. 19 Monkey Business Images/Shutterstock.com; p. 23 3D character/Shutterstock.com; cover graphics blackpencil/Shutterstock.com.